MW01298326

THIS JOURNAL
BELONGS TO:

PROGRESS TRACKER

Week	Weight	Neck	Chest	Upper arm	Waist	Hips	Thigh	Calf
1								
2								
3								
4								
5								
6								
7								
8								
9								
10								
11								
12								
13								
14								

DAILY JOURNAL

Week

Date

Weight   Ketones   Sleep

Time	Food or beverage and serving	Carbs (g)	Protein (g)	Fat (g)	Calories
	Total				

NOTES (e.g. about energy level, non-scale victories, meal ideas)

DAILY JOURNAL

Week

Date

Weight   Ketones   Sleep

Time	Food or beverage and serving	Carbs (g)	Protein (g)	Fat (g)	Calories
	Total				

NOTES (e.g. about energy level, non-scale victories, meal ideas)

DAILY JOURNAL

Week

Date

Weight   Ketones   Sleep

Time	Food or beverage and serving	Carbs (g)	Protein (g)	Fat (g)	Calories
	Total				

NOTES (e.g. about energy level, non-scale victories, meal ideas)

DAILY JOURNAL

Week _____
Date _____

Weight _____   Ketones _____   Sleep _____

Time	Food or beverage and serving	Carbs (g)	Protein (g)	Fat (g)	Calories
	Total				

NOTES (e.g. about energy level, non-scale victories, meal ideas)

DAILY JOURNAL

Week

Date

Weight   Ketones   Sleep

Time	Food or beverage and serving	Carbs (g)	Protein (g)	Fat (g)	Calories
	Total				

NOTES (e.g. about energy level, non-scale victories, meal ideas)

DAILY JOURNAL

Week [ ]
Date [ ]

Weight [ ]   Ketones [ ]   Sleep [ ]

Time	Food or beverage and serving	Carbs (g)	Protein (g)	Fat (g)	Calories
	Total				

NOTES (e.g. about energy level, non-scale victories, meal ideas)

DAILY JOURNAL

Week

Date

Weight   Ketones   Sleep

Time	Food or beverage and serving	Carbs (g)	Protein (g)	Fat (g)	Calories
		Total			

NOTES (e.g. about energy level, non-scale victories, meal ideas)

DAILY JOURNAL

Week

Date

Weight   Ketones   Sleep

Time	Food or beverage and serving	Carbs (g)	Protein (g)	Fat (g)	Calories
	Total				

NOTES (e.g. about energy level, non-scale victories, meal ideas)

DAILY JOURNAL

Week

Date

Weight   Ketones   Sleep

Time	Food or beverage and serving	Carbs (g)	Protein (g)	Fat (g)	Calories
	Total				

NOTES (e.g. about energy level, non-scale victories, meal ideas)

DAILY JOURNAL

Week ____

Date ____

Weight _____ Ketones _____ Sleep _____

Time	Food or beverage and serving	Carbs (g)	Protein (g)	Fat (g)	Calories
	Total				

NOTES (e.g. about energy level, non-scale victories, meal ideas)

DAILY JOURNAL

Week

Date

Weight   Ketones   Sleep

Time	Food or beverage and serving	Carbs (g)	Protein (g)	Fat (g)	Calories
	Total				

NOTES (e.g. about energy level, non-scale victories, meal ideas)

DAILY JOURNAL

Week

Date

Weight   Ketones   Sleep

Time	Food or beverage and serving	Carbs (g)	Protein (g)	Fat (g)	Calories
	Total				

NOTES (e.g. about energy level, non-scale victories, meal ideas)

DAILY JOURNAL

Week
Date

Weight   Ketones   Sleep

Time	Food or beverage and serving	Carbs (g)	Protein (g)	Fat (g)	Calories
	Total				

NOTES (e.g. about energy level, non-scale victories, meal ideas)

DAILY JOURNAL

Week

Date

Weight _____ Ketones _____ Sleep _____

Time	Food or beverage and serving	Carbs (g)	Protein (g)	Fat (g)	Calories
	Total				

NOTES (e.g. about energy level, non-scale victories, meal ideas)

DAILY JOURNAL

Week

Date

Weight _____ Ketones _____ Sleep _____

Time	Food or beverage and serving	Carbs (g)	Protein (g)	Fat (g)	Calories
	Total				

NOTES (e.g. about energy level, non-scale victories, meal ideas)

DAILY JOURNAL

Week
Date

Weight _____ Ketones _____ Sleep _____

Time	Food or beverage and serving	Carbs (g)	Protein (g)	Fat (g)	Calories
	Total				

NOTES (e.g. about energy level, non-scale victories, meal ideas)

DAILY JOURNAL

Week

Date

Weight   Ketones   Sleep

Time	Food or beverage and serving	Carbs (g)	Protein (g)	Fat (g)	Calories
	Total				

NOTES (e.g. about energy level, non-scale victories, meal ideas)

DAILY JOURNAL

Week

Date

Weight   Ketones   Sleep

Time	Food or beverage and serving	Carbs (g)	Protein (g)	Fat (g)	Calories
	Total				

NOTES (e.g. about energy level, non-scale victories, meal ideas)

DAILY JOURNAL

Week
Date

Weight   Ketones   Sleep

Time	Food or beverage and serving	Carbs (g)	Protein (g)	Fat (g)	Calories
	Total				

NOTES (e.g. about energy level, non-scale victories, meal ideas)

DAILY JOURNAL

Week
Date

Weight   Ketones   Sleep

Time	Food or beverage and serving	Carbs (g)	Protein (g)	Fat (g)	Calories
	Total				

NOTES (e.g. about energy level, non-scale victories, meal ideas)

DAILY JOURNAL

Week

Date

Weight   Ketones   Sleep

Time	Food or beverage and serving	Carbs (g)	Protein (g)	Fat (g)	Calories
	Total				

NOTES (e.g. about energy level, non-scale victories, meal ideas)

DAILY JOURNAL

Week
Date

Weight   Ketones   Sleep

Time	Food or beverage and serving	Carbs (g)	Protein (g)	Fat (g)	Calories
	Total				

NOTES (e.g. about energy level, non-scale victories, meal ideas)

DAILY JOURNAL

Week

Date

Weight _____ Ketones _____ Sleep _____

Time	Food or beverage and serving	Carbs (g)	Protein (g)	Fat (g)	Calories
			Total				

NOTES (e.g. about energy level, non-scale victories, meal ideas)

DAILY JOURNAL

Week

Date

Weight   Ketones   Sleep

Time	Food or beverage and serving	Carbs (g)	Protein (g)	Fat (g)	Calories
	Total				

NOTES (e.g. about energy level, non-scale victories, meal ideas)

DAILY JOURNAL

Week _____
Date _____

Weight _____   Ketones _____   Sleep _____

Time	Food or beverage and serving	Carbs (g)	Protein (g)	Fat (g)	Calories
	Total				

NOTES (e.g. about energy level, non-scale victories, meal ideas)

DAILY JOURNAL

Week
Date

Weight   Ketones   Sleep

Time	Food or beverage and serving	Carbs (g)	Protein (g)	Fat (g)	Calories
	Total				

NOTES (e.g. about energy level, non-scale victories, meal ideas)

DAILY JOURNAL

Week

Date

Weight _____ Ketones _____ Sleep _____

Time	Food or beverage and serving	Carbs (g)	Protein (g)	Fat (g)	Calories
	Total				

NOTES (e.g. about energy level, non-scale victories, meal ideas)

DAILY JOURNAL

Week

Date

Weight   Ketones   Sleep

Time	Food or beverage and serving	Carbs (g)	Protein (g)	Fat (g)	Calories
	Total				

NOTES (e.g. about energy level, non-scale victories, meal ideas)

DAILY JOURNAL

Week

Date

Weight   Ketones   Sleep

Time	Food or beverage and serving	Carbs (g)	Protein (g)	Fat (g)	Calories
	Total				

NOTES (e.g. about energy level, non-scale victories, meal ideas)

DAILY JOURNAL

Week

Date

Weight   Ketones   Sleep

Time	Food or beverage and serving	Carbs (g)	Protein (g)	Fat (g)	Calories
	Total				

NOTES (e.g. about energy level, non-scale victories, meal ideas)

DAILY JOURNAL

Week

Date

Weight _____ Ketones _____ Sleep _____

Time	Food or beverage and serving	Carbs (g)	Protein (g)	Fat (g)	Calories
	Total				

NOTES (e.g. about energy level, non-scale victories, meal ideas)

DAILY JOURNAL

Week

Date

Weight   Ketones   Sleep

Time	Food or beverage and serving	Carbs (g)	Protein (g)	Fat (g)	Calories
	Total				

NOTES (e.g. about energy level, non-scale victories, meal ideas)

DAILY JOURNAL

Week

Date

Weight   Ketones   Sleep

Time	Food or beverage and serving	Carbs (g)	Protein (g)	Fat (g)	Calories
		Total			

NOTES (e.g. about energy level, non-scale victories, meal ideas)

DAILY JOURNAL

Week
Date

Weight   Ketones   Sleep

Time	Food or beverage and serving	Carbs (g)	Protein (g)	Fat (g)	Calories
	Total				

NOTES (e.g. about energy level, non-scale victories, meal ideas)

DAILY JOURNAL

Week

Date

Weight   Ketones   Sleep

Time	Food or beverage and serving	Carbs (g)	Protein (g)	Fat (g)	Calories
	Total				

NOTES (e.g. about energy level, non-scale victories, meal ideas)

DAILY JOURNAL

Week

Date

Weight   Ketones   Sleep

Time	Food or beverage and serving	Carbs (g)	Protein (g)	Fat (g)	Calories
		Total			

NOTES (e.g. about energy level, non-scale victories, meal ideas)

DAILY JOURNAL

Week _____
Date _____

Weight _____   Ketones _____   Sleep _____

Time	Food or beverage and serving	Carbs (g)	Protein (g)	Fat (g)	Calories
	Total				

NOTES (e.g. about energy level, non-scale victories, meal ideas)

DAILY JOURNAL

Week
Date

Weight   Ketones   Sleep

Time	Food or beverage and serving	Carbs (g)	Protein (g)	Fat (g)	Calories
	Total				

NOTES (e.g. about energy level, non-scale victories, meal ideas)

DAILY JOURNAL

Week

Date

Weight _____ Ketones _____ Sleep _____

Time	Food or beverage and serving	Carbs (g)	Protein (g)	Fat (g)	Calories
	Total				

NOTES (e.g. about energy level, non-scale victories, meal ideas)

DAILY JOURNAL

Week
Date

Weight   Ketones   Sleep

Time	Food or beverage and serving	Carbs (g)	Protein (g)	Fat (g)	Calories
	Total				

NOTES (e.g. about energy level, non-scale victories, meal ideas)

DAILY JOURNAL

Week

Date

Weight   Ketones   Sleep

Time	Food or beverage and serving	Carbs (g)	Protein (g)	Fat (g)	Calories
	Total				

NOTES (e.g. about energy level, non-scale victories, meal ideas)

DAILY JOURNAL

Week

Date

Weight _____ Ketones _____ Sleep _____

Time	Food or beverage and serving	Carbs (g)	Protein (g)	Fat (g)	Calories
	Total				

NOTES (e.g. about energy level, non-scale victories, meal ideas)

DAILY JOURNAL

Week
Date

Weight   Ketones   Sleep

Time	Food or beverage and serving	Carbs (g)	Protein (g)	Fat (g)	Calories
	Total				

NOTES (e.g. about energy level, non-scale victories, meal ideas)

DAILY JOURNAL

Week

Date

Weight   Ketones   Sleep

Time	Food or beverage and serving	Carbs (g)	Protein (g)	Fat (g)	Calories
	Total				

NOTES (e.g. about energy level, non-scale victories, meal ideas)

DAILY JOURNAL

Week _____
Date _____

Weight _____   Ketones _____   Sleep _____

Time	Food or beverage and serving	Carbs (g)	Protein (g)	Fat (g)	Calories
	Total				

NOTES (e.g. about energy level, non-scale victories, meal ideas)

DAILY JOURNAL

Week

Date

Weight   Ketones   Sleep

Time	Food or beverage and serving	Carbs (g)	Protein (g)	Fat (g)	Calories
Total					

NOTES (e.g. about energy level, non-scale victories, meal ideas)

DAILY JOURNAL

Week

Date

Weight   Ketones   Sleep

Time	Food or beverage and serving	Carbs (g)	Protein (g)	Fat (g)	Calories
	Total				

NOTES (e.g. about energy level, non-scale victories, meal ideas)

DAILY JOURNAL

Week
Date

Weight   Ketones   Sleep

Time	Food or beverage and serving	Carbs (g)	Protein (g)	Fat (g)	Calories
	Total				

NOTES (e.g. about energy level, non-scale victories, meal ideas)

DAILY JOURNAL

Week

Date

Weight _____ Ketones _____ Sleep _____

Time	Food or beverage and serving	Carbs (g)	Protein (g)	Fat (g)	Calories
	Total				

NOTES (e.g. about energy level, non-scale victories, meal ideas)

DAILY JOURNAL

Week
Date

Weight   Ketones   Sleep

Time	Food or beverage and serving	Carbs (g)	Protein (g)	Fat (g)	Calories
	Total				

NOTES (e.g. about energy level, non-scale victories, meal ideas)

DAILY JOURNAL

Week

Date

Weight _____ Ketones _____ Sleep _____

Time	Food or beverage and serving	Carbs (g)	Protein (g)	Fat (g)	Calories
	Total				

NOTES (e.g. about energy level, non-scale victories, meal ideas)

DAILY JOURNAL

Week

Date

Weight   Ketones   Sleep

Time	Food or beverage and serving	Carbs (g)	Protein (g)	Fat (g)	Calories
	Total				

NOTES (e.g. about energy level, non-scale victories, meal ideas)

DAILY JOURNAL

Week
Date

Weight _____ Ketones _____ Sleep _____

Time	Food or beverage and serving	Carbs (g)	Protein (g)	Fat (g)	Calories
	Total				

NOTES (e.g. about energy level, non-scale victories, meal ideas)

DAILY JOURNAL

Week
Date

Weight   Ketones   Sleep

Time	Food or beverage and serving	Carbs (g)	Protein (g)	Fat (g)	Calories
	Total				

NOTES (e.g. about energy level, non-scale victories, meal ideas)

DAILY JOURNAL

Week

Date

Weight   Ketones   Sleep

Time	Food or beverage and serving	Carbs (g)	Protein (g)	Fat (g)	Calories
	Total				

NOTES (e.g. about energy level, non-scale victories, meal ideas)

DAILY JOURNAL

Week
Date

Weight   Ketones   Sleep

Time	Food or beverage and serving	Carbs (g)	Protein (g)	Fat (g)	Calories
	Total				

NOTES (e.g. about energy level, non-scale victories, meal ideas)

DAILY JOURNAL

Week

Date

Weight   Ketones   Sleep

Time	Food or beverage and serving	Carbs (g)	Protein (g)	Fat (g)	Calories
	Total				

NOTES (e.g. about energy level, non-scale victories, meal ideas)

DAILY JOURNAL

Week
Date

Weight ____ Ketones ____ Sleep ____

Time	Food or beverage and serving	Carbs (g)	Protein (g)	Fat (g)	Calories
	Total				

NOTES (e.g. about energy level, non-scale victories, meal ideas)

DAILY JOURNAL

Week

Date

Weight   Ketones   Sleep

Time	Food or beverage and serving	Carbs (g)	Protein (g)	Fat (g)	Calories
	Total				

NOTES (e.g. about energy level, non-scale victories, meal ideas)

DAILY JOURNAL

Week

Date

Weight   Ketones   Sleep

Time	Food or beverage and serving	Carbs (g)	Protein (g)	Fat (g)	Calories
		Total			

NOTES (e.g. about energy level, non-scale victories, meal ideas)

DAILY JOURNAL

Week

Date

Weight   Ketones   Sleep

Time	Food or beverage and serving	Carbs (g)	Protein (g)	Fat (g)	Calories
	Total				

NOTES (e.g. about energy level, non-scale victories, meal ideas)

DAILY JOURNAL

Week

Date

Weight   Ketones   Sleep

Time	Food or beverage and serving	Carbs (g)	Protein (g)	Fat (g)	Calories
	Total				

NOTES (e.g. about energy level, non-scale victories, meal ideas)

DAILY JOURNAL

Week

Date

Weight _____ Ketones _____ Sleep _____

Time	Food or beverage and serving	Carbs (g)	Protein (g)	Fat (g)	Calories
	Total				

NOTES (e.g. about energy level, non-scale victories, meal ideas)

DAILY JOURNAL

Week

Date

Weight   Ketones   Sleep

Time	Food or beverage and serving	Carbs (g)	Protein (g)	Fat (g)	Calories
	Total				

NOTES (e.g. about energy level, non-scale victories, meal ideas)

DAILY JOURNAL

Week

Date

Weight _____ Ketones _____ Sleep _____

Time	Food or beverage and serving	Carbs (g)	Protein (g)	Fat (g)	Calories
	Total				

NOTES (e.g. about energy level, non-scale victories, meal ideas)

DAILY JOURNAL

Week

Date

Weight   Ketones   Sleep

Time	Food or beverage and serving	Carbs (g)	Protein (g)	Fat (g)	Calories
	Total				

NOTES (e.g. about energy level, non-scale victories, meal ideas)

DAILY JOURNAL

Week

Date

Weight _____ Ketones _____ Sleep _____

Time	Food or beverage and serving	Carbs (g)	Protein (g)	Fat (g)	Calories
	Total				

NOTES (e.g. about energy level, non-scale victories, meal ideas)

DAILY JOURNAL

Week

Date

Weight

Ketones

Sleep

Time	Food or beverage and serving	Carbs (g)	Protein (g)	Fat (g)	Calories
	Total				

NOTES (e.g. about energy level, non-scale victories, meal ideas)

DAILY JOURNAL

Week
Date

Weight _____   Ketones _____   Sleep _____

Time	Food or beverage and serving	Carbs (g)	Protein (g)	Fat (g)	Calories
	Total				

NOTES (e.g. about energy level, non-scale victories, meal ideas)

DAILY JOURNAL

Week
Date

Weight ▢ Ketones ▢ Sleep ▢

Time	Food or beverage and serving	Carbs (g)	Protein (g)	Fat (g)	Calories
	Total				

NOTES (e.g. about energy level, non-scale victories, meal ideas)

DAILY JOURNAL

Week

Date

Weight _____ Ketones _____ Sleep _____

Time	Food or beverage and serving	Carbs (g)	Protein (g)	Fat (g)	Calories
	Total				

NOTES (e.g. about energy level, non-scale victories, meal ideas)

DAILY JOURNAL

Week

Date

Weight   Ketones   Sleep

Time	Food or beverage and serving	Carbs (g)	Protein (g)	Fat (g)	Calories
	Total				

NOTES (e.g. about energy level, non-scale victories, meal ideas)

DAILY JOURNAL

Week

Date

Weight   Ketones   Sleep

Time	Food or beverage and serving	Carbs (g)	Protein (g)	Fat (g)	Calories
	Total				

NOTES (e.g. about energy level, non-scale victories, meal ideas)

DAILY JOURNAL

Week
Date

Weight   Ketones   Sleep

Time	Food or beverage and serving	Carbs (g)	Protein (g)	Fat (g)	Calories
	Total				

NOTES (e.g. about energy level, non-scale victories, meal ideas)

DAILY JOURNAL

Week
Date

Weight   Ketones   Sleep

Time	Food or beverage and serving	Carbs (g)	Protein (g)	Fat (g)	Calories
	Total				

NOTES (e.g. about energy level, non-scale victories, meal ideas)

DAILY JOURNAL

Week

Date

Weight   Ketones   Sleep

Time	Food or beverage and serving	Carbs (g)	Protein (g)	Fat (g)	Calories
	Total				

NOTES (e.g. about energy level, non-scale victories, meal ideas)

DAILY JOURNAL

Week

Date

Weight   Ketones   Sleep

Time	Food or beverage and serving	Carbs (g)	Protein (g)	Fat (g)	Calories
	Total				

NOTES (e.g. about energy level, non-scale victories, meal ideas)

DAILY JOURNAL

Week
Date

Weight   Ketones   Sleep

Time	Food or beverage and serving	Carbs (g)	Protein (g)	Fat (g)	Calories
	Total				

NOTES (e.g. about energy level, non-scale victories, meal ideas)

DAILY JOURNAL

Week
Date

Weight   Ketones   Sleep

Time	Food or beverage and serving	Carbs (g)	Protein (g)	Fat (g)	Calories
	Total				

NOTES (e.g. about energy level, non-scale victories, meal ideas)

DAILY JOURNAL

Week
Date

Weight   Ketones   Sleep

Time	Food or beverage and serving	Carbs (g)	Protein (g)	Fat (g)	Calories
	Total				

NOTES (e.g. about energy level, non-scale victories, meal ideas)

DAILY JOURNAL

Week
Date

Weight   Ketones   Sleep

Time	Food or beverage and serving	Carbs (g)	Protein (g)	Fat (g)	Calories
	Total				

NOTES (e.g. about energy level, non-scale victories, meal ideas)

DAILY JOURNAL

Week

Date

Weight   Ketones   Sleep

Time	Food or beverage and serving	Carbs (g)	Protein (g)	Fat (g)	Calories
	Total				

NOTES (e.g. about energy level, non-scale victories, meal ideas)

DAILY JOURNAL

Week

Date

Weight   Ketones   Sleep

Time	Food or beverage and serving	Carbs (g)	Protein (g)	Fat (g)	Calories
	Total				

NOTES (e.g. about energy level, non-scale victories, meal ideas)

DAILY JOURNAL

Week

Date

Weight   Ketones   Sleep

Time	Food or beverage and serving	Carbs (g)	Protein (g)	Fat (g)	Calories
	Total				

NOTES (e.g. about energy level, non-scale victories, meal ideas)

DAILY JOURNAL

Week

Date

Weight   Ketones   Sleep

Time	Food or beverage and serving	Carbs (g)	Protein (g)	Fat (g)	Calories
	Total				

NOTES (e.g. about energy level, non-scale victories, meal ideas)

DAILY JOURNAL

Week

Date

Weight   Ketones   Sleep

Time	Food or beverage and serving	Carbs (g)	Protein (g)	Fat (g)	Calories
	Total				

NOTES (e.g. about energy level, non-scale victories, meal ideas)

DAILY JOURNAL

Week
Date

Weight _____ Ketones _____ Sleep _____

Time	Food or beverage and serving	Carbs (g)	Protein (g)	Fat (g)	Calories
	Total				

NOTES (e.g. about energy level, non-scale victories, meal ideas)

DAILY JOURNAL

Week

Date

Weight   Ketones   Sleep

Time	Food or beverage and serving	Carbs (g)	Protein (g)	Fat (g)	Calories
	Total				

NOTES (e.g. about energy level, non-scale victories, meal ideas)

DAILY JOURNAL

Week

Date

Weight   Ketones   Sleep

Time	Food or beverage and serving	Carbs (g)	Protein (g)	Fat (g)	Calories
	Total				

NOTES (e.g. about energy level, non-scale victories, meal ideas)

DAILY JOURNAL

Week

Date

Weight   Ketones   Sleep

Time	Food or beverage and serving	Carbs (g)	Protein (g)	Fat (g)	Calories
	Total				

NOTES (e.g. about energy level, non-scale victories, meal ideas)

DAILY JOURNAL

Week

Date

Weight   Ketones   Sleep

Time	Food or beverage and serving	Carbs (g)	Protein (g)	Fat (g)	Calories
	Total				

NOTES (e.g. about energy level, non-scale victories, meal ideas)

DAILY JOURNAL

Week ____

Date ____

Weight ____   Ketones ____   Sleep ____

Time	Food or beverage and serving	Carbs (g)	Protein (g)	Fat (g)	Calories
	Total				

NOTES (e.g. about energy level, non-scale victories, meal ideas)

DAILY JOURNAL

Week

Date

Weight   Ketones   Sleep

Time	Food or beverage and serving	Carbs (g)	Protein (g)	Fat (g)	Calories
	Total				

NOTES (e.g. about energy level, non-scale victories, meal ideas)

DAILY JOURNAL

Week

Date

Weight | Ketones | Sleep

Time	Food or beverage and serving	Carbs (g)	Protein (g)	Fat (g)	Calories
	Total				

NOTES (e.g. about energy level, non-scale victories, meal ideas)

DAILY JOURNAL

Week ▮▮▮

Date ▮▮▮

Weight ▮▮▮ Ketones ▮▮▮ Sleep ▮▮▮

Time	Food or beverage and serving	Carbs (g)	Protein (g)	Fat (g)	Calories
	Total				

NOTES (e.g. about energy level, non-scale victories, meal ideas)

DAILY JOURNAL

Week ▒▒▒▒
Date ▒▒▒▒

Weight ▒▒▒▒ Ketones ▒▒▒▒ Sleep ▒▒▒▒

Time	Food or beverage and serving	Carbs (g)	Protein (g)	Fat (g)	Calories
		Total				

NOTES (e.g. about energy level, non-scale victories, meal ideas)

DAILY JOURNAL

Week

Date

Weight   Ketones   Sleep

Time	Food or beverage and serving	Carbs (g)	Protein (g)	Fat (g)	Calories
	Total				

NOTES (e.g. about energy level, non-scale victories, meal ideas)

DAILY JOURNAL

Week

Date

Weight   Ketones   Sleep

Time	Food or beverage and serving	Carbs (g)	Protein (g)	Fat (g)	Calories
	Total				

NOTES (e.g. about energy level, non-scale victories, meal ideas)

Made in United States
Orlando, FL
11 November 2022

24416680R00057